Intermi
Fasting For Women
Over 60

The Ultimate Guide to Effortlessly Lose
Weight, Slow Aging, and Detoxify Your Body

Lara R. Clark

Table of Contents

INTRODUCTION

As we travel along the road of life, our physical bodies change and our health requirements transform. For many women over sixty years old, keeping healthy can be a challenge but it is also more important than ever before. And this is where intermittent fasting can play a vital role. Intermittent fasting is not just about losing weight, though it undeniably contributes to that. It means a chance for your body to reset and rejuvenate thereby supporting general well-being and health. Intermittent fasting could be advantageous in some ways:

- Better Metabolism: As we grow older, our metabolism might slow down significantly. Intermittent fasting helps get your metabolism going again allowing you to shed pounds and get more vibrant.

- Improved Hormonal Balance: There are many hormonal changes experienced with age; these alterations may result in mood swings as well as fluctuations in weight among other things. It has been suggested that the use of intermittent fasting could restore hormone balance leading to a steadier emotional state and overall improved health condition.

- Improved Brain Functioning: Some research studies have revealed that there exists a connection between intermittent fasting and brain well-being which includes memory consolidation as well as enhanced attention span. This becomes even more critical when one gets aged but still wants their cognitive ability to remain intact.
- Longer Lifespan: Preliminary evidence suggests that intermittent fasting may prolong life expectancy, reduce cardiovascular diseases

How This Book Can Help You Achieve Your Health Goals

At this point, you may be wondering how to start intermittent fasting and make it work for you. That's where this book fits in. It is not just a cookbook with lots of recipes and meal plans. Instead, it offers an all-inclusive guide customized for ladies over the age of 60 who wish to use intermittent fasting as their path toward healthier lives.

This book includes:

- Practical Advice: Learn how to incorporate intermittent fasting safely into your lifestyle, including tips on overcoming common challenges.
- Nutritional Guidance: Explore the best foods to eat during this period to maintain your well-being.
- Recipes and Meal Plans: Enjoy various mouthwatering meals full of nutrition specifically formulated for older women who are following an intermittent diet program

Understanding Intermittent Fasting: The Basics

Initially, it may sound impossible to go about when starting in the game of intermittent fasting; however, it is simple enough at some point. This involves alternating periods of eating and fasting. The most popular technique is known as 16/8 fast which was popularized by Martin Berkhan, whereby fasting takes 16 hours while eating takes place within eight hours.

During the fasting period, your body switches to burning stored fat for energy, which can lead to weight loss and other health benefits. And don't worry, fasting doesn't mean starving yourself. You can still eat plenty of nutritious foods during your eating window to support your health and well-being.

GETTING STARTED WITH INTERMITTENT FASTING

How to Begin Intermittent Fasting Safely

It takes an act of courage towards good health to start on the path of intermittent fasting. It is a journey that begins with self-awareness and compassion, recognizing that it is a transformative process that requires time and patience. Here are some baby steps to get you started safely with intermittent fasting.

1. Take Your Time: Slowly increase your fasting period over time. A 12-hour fast can be extended gradually into 16 or even 18 hours. Adjust according to what your body tells you.

2. Stay Hydrated: While fasting, hydration is very important. Make sure you drink enough water, herbal tea, and other noncaloric beverages since they will help reduce hunger pangs as well as keep your skin hydrated.

3. Pick Nutrient-dense Food: When breaking your fast focus eat nutrient-packed foods that will fuel up your body Ensure each of the meals contains lots of fruits, vegetables whole grains lean proteins, and healthy fats.

4. Check with Yourself: Find out how you feel during this period when not eating much food at all. If one feels faint or light-headed or excessively hungry then it might result from a fasting schedule which could have changed for example by having a small balanced meal instead

5. Be Patient and Kind to Yourself: Remember, intermittent fasting is a lifestyle change, not a quick fix. It's okay to have days where you struggle or slip up. Be gentle with yourself and keep moving forward.

Finding the Right Fasting Schedule for You

Time, discovery of self, and prioritizing the body's needs are what it takes to discover the right fasting schedule. It is a matter of choosing the most appropriate health measure that suits your unique health requirements. Nonetheless, sometimes it might be hard to identify the best fasting schedule for you. Here are steps that can help you find the right fasting schedule for yourself.

1. Know Your Objectives: Why do you want to try intermittent fasting? Do you want to lose weight, have more energy, or just promote your overall health? Understanding your objectives better will enable you to match them with an ideal intermittent fasting program.

2. Think About Your Lifestyle: Think about how an intermittent fast could work within your routine day after day. Are there particular times when you feel more hungry or vibrant? Going by this creates conducive conditions that assist in sticking to one's natural clock.

3. Try Different Schedules: There are many types of fasts available like 16:8 fasts, 5:2 fasts, and alternate-day fasts among others. You can experiment with different schedules until find out which one works best for you as a person who's trying to get into shape through the intermittent fasting method. Pay

attention to how you feel during and after periods of fasting so this way, you can tell which schedule seems practical for you.

4. Nurture Yourself: Most of the time we undermine our body's capabilities anyway; we should ask them first since they know us well enough and know where they've been taken wrong by them too often before taking any action plan.

5. Be Flexible: Your fasting schedule may need to change over time as your body and lifestyle change. Be open to adjusting your schedule as needed to ensure it continues to support your health goals.

Finding the right fasting schedule for you is a journey, one that requires patience, self-awareness, and a willingness to listen to your body. By understanding your goals, considering your lifestyle, experimenting with different schedules, listening to your body, and being flexible, you can find a fasting schedule that supports your health and well-being.

Tips for Success: Overcoming Common Challenges

You must remember that you are not alone in this new path of eating. Other people who trod on this path before you have had experiences that will help you a lot and give valuable insights. Below are some tips to overcome the most common challenges and be successful with intermittent fasting.

1. Stay Hydrated: Drink adequate amounts of water, and non-caloric drinks like herbal tea, etc. during your fasting periods to prevent dehydration and curb hunger.

2. Listen to Your Body: Pay attention to how you feel during your fasting periods. Feeling lightheaded, dizzy, or very hungry could be an indication that it is time for a fast adjustment or having a small balanced meal.

3. Start Slowly: Beginners should introduce intermittent fasting gradually by increasing the duration of their fasting periods. This gentle approach helps the body adapt better, reducing the chances of intense cravings or hunger pangs.

4. Focus on Nutrient-Dense Foods: Break your fast by consuming foods rich in nutrients that support the body's well-being; fruits, vegetables, whole grains, lean proteins, and healthy fats ought to come first since they will leave one feeling full and energized at the same time.

5. Planning: Beforehand: Plan your meals and snacks to stick to your fasting timetable. Make some healthy food and snacks for easy pick up while in the window of eating so that you won't be tempted to take junk food.

6. Stay Positive: While fasting can be hard at times, keeping a good attitude will assist you overcome any hurdles you face. Remember why you started intermittent fasting and how it could be beneficial to your health and well-being.

Note that intermittent fasting is a journey with ups and downs along the way it's okay to experience them. Hydrating yourself, listening to your body, going slow, focusing on nutrient-dense foods, planning, and thinking positively are among the ways through which you can surmount these common challenges and succeed with the concept of intermittent fasting.

CHAPTER 1: BREAKFAST

Apple Cinnamon Oatmeal

INGREDIENTS:

- 1/2 cup rolled oats

- 1 cup almond milk

- 1 small apple, diced

- 1/2 teaspoon cinnamon

- 1 tablespoon chopped nuts (optional)

INSTRUCTION:

1. Cook over medium heat, stirring occasionally, until oats are tender, about 5 minutes.
2. Stir in diced apple and cinnamon.
3. Cook for an additional 2-3 minutes, until apple is soft.
4. Remove from heat and let cool slightly before serving. Sprinkle with chopped nuts if desired.

Greek Yogurt Parfait with Berries

INGREDIENTS:

- 1 cup Greek yogurt
- 1/2 cup mixed berries (such as strawberries, blueberries, and raspberries)
- 2 tablespoons honey
- 1/4 cup granola

INSTRUCTIONS:

1. In a glass, layer Greek yogurt, mixed berries, honey, and granola.
2. Repeat layers until ingredients are used up.
3. Serve immediately.

Veggie Omelet with Spinach and Tomatoes

INGREDIENTS:

- 2 eggs

- 1/4 cup chopped spinach
- 1/4 cup diced tomatoes
- 1/4 cup shredded cheese (optional)
- Salt and pepper to taste

INSTRUCTIONS:

1. In a bowl, whisk together eggs, spinach, tomatoes, cheese, salt, and pepper.
2. Pour mixture into a heated, greased skillet.
3. Cook until the eggs are set, about 3-4 minutes.
4. Fold the omelet in half and serve hot.

Chia Seed Pudding with Almond Milk

INGREDIENTS:

- 1/4 cup chia seeds
- 1 cup almond milk
- 1 tablespoon honey or maple syrup
- 1/2 teaspoon vanilla extract
- Fresh fruit for topping

INSTRUCTIONS:

1. In a bowl, combine chia seeds, almond milk, honey or maple syrup, and vanilla extract.
2. Stir well to combine.
3. Cover and refrigerate for at least 2 hours, or overnight.
4. Serve chilled, topped with fresh fruit.

Avocado Toast with Poached Egg

INGREDIENTS:

- 1 slice whole grain bread, toasted
- 1/2 avocado, mashed
- 1 poached egg
- Salt and pepper to taste

INSTRUCTIONS:

1. Spread mashed avocado on toasted bread.
2. Top with a poached egg.

3. Season with salt and pepper to taste.

Blueberry Banana Smoothie

INGREDIENTS:

- 1/2 cup blueberries
- 1/2 banana
- 1/2 cup Greek yogurt
- 1/2 cup almond milk
- 1 tablespoon honey or maple syrup

INSTRUCTIONS:

1. Combine blueberries, banana, Greek yogurt, almond milk, and honey or maple syrup in a blender.
2. Blend until smooth.
3. Pour into a glass and serve immediately.

Whole Grain Pancakes with Maple Syrup

INGREDIENTS:

- 1/2 cup whole grain flour

- 1/2 teaspoon baking powder
- 1/2 cup almond milk
- 1 egg
- 1 tablespoon maple syrup
- 1/2 teaspoon vanilla extract

INSTRUCTIONS:

1. In a bowl, whisk together flour and baking powder.
2. In a separate bowl, whisk together almond milk, egg, maple syrup, and vanilla extract.
3. Pour wet ingredients into dry ingredients and stir until just combined.
4. Heat a greased skillet over medium heat.
5. Pour batter onto skillet to form pancakes.
6. Cook until bubbles form on the surface, then flip and cook until golden brown.
7. Serve hot with maple syrup.

Breakfast Burrito with Black Beans and Salsa

INGREDIENTS:

- 1 whole grain tortilla
- 1/4 cup black beans
- 2 eggs, scrambled
- 2 tablespoons salsa
- 1/4 avocado, sliced

INSTRUCTIONS:

1. Heat the tortilla in a skillet over medium heat.
2. Spread black beans on the tortilla.
3. Top with scrambled eggs, salsa, and avocado slices.
4. Roll up the tortilla to form a burrito.

Quinoa Breakfast Bowl with Nuts and Seeds

INGREDIENTS:

- 1/2 cup cooked quinoa

- 1/4 cup Greek yogurt
- 1 tablespoon honey or maple syrup
- 1 tablespoon chopped nuts
- 1 tablespoon mixed seeds (such as chia seeds, flaxseeds, and pumpkin seeds)

INSTRUCTIONS:

1. In a bowl, combine cooked quinoa, Greek yogurt, honey or maple syrup, nuts, and seeds.
2. Stir well to combine.
3. Serve warm or chilled.

Sweet Potato Hash with Turkey Sausage

INGREDIENTS:

- 1 sweet potato, diced
- 1/4 onion, diced
- 1/4 bell pepper, diced
- 2 turkey sausage links, sliced
- 1/2 teaspoon smoked paprika

- Salt and pepper to taste

INSTRUCTIONS:

1. In a skillet, heat olive oil over medium heat.
2. Add sweet potato, onion, bell pepper, and turkey sausage.
3. Season with smoked paprika, salt, and pepper.
4. Cook, stirring occasionally, until the sweet potato is tender and the sausage is cooked through.
5. Serve hot.

CHAPTER 2: APPETIZERS & SNACKS

Guacamole with Baked Tortilla Chips

GUACAMOLE INGREDIENTS:

- 2 ripe avocados
- 1/4 cup diced red onion
- 1/4 cup chopped fresh cilantro
- 1 small jalapeño, seeded and minced
- Juice of 1 lime
- Salt and pepper to taste

BAKED TORTILLA CHIPS INGREDIENTS:

- 4 whole grain tortillas

- Cooking spray
- Salt to taste

GUACAMOLE INSTRUCTIONS:

1. Cut avocados in half, remove the pit, and scoop the flesh into a bowl.

2. Mash the avocado with a fork until smooth, but still slightly chunky.

3. Stir in red onion, cilantro, jalapeño, lime juice, salt, and pepper.

BAKED TORTILLA CHIPS INSTRUCTIONS:

1. Preheat oven to 350°F (175°C).
2. Cut tortillas into wedges and place them on a baking sheet.
3. Spray both sides of the tortilla wedges with cooking spray and sprinkle with salt.
4. Bake for 10-12 minutes, or until crispy and golden brown.

5. Serve the guacamole with the baked tortilla chips for a delicious snack or appetizer.

Hummus with Crudites

INGREDIENTS:

- 1 can (15 ounces) chickpeas, drained and rinsed
- 2 cloves garlic, minced
- 3 tablespoons tahini
- Juice of 1 lemon
- 2 tablespoons olive oil
- Salt and pepper to taste
- Assorted crudites (such as carrots, cucumbers, bell peppers, and cherry tomatoes) for dipping

INSTRUCTIONS:

1. In a food processor, combine chickpeas, garlic, tahini, lemon juice, olive oil, salt, and pepper.
2. Blend until smooth, adding water as needed to achieve desired consistency.
3. Serve hummus with crudites for dipping.

Spicy Edamame

INGREDIENTS:

- 1 pound frozen edamame in pods
- 2 tablespoons olive oil
- 1 teaspoon chili powder
- 1/2 teaspoon garlic powder
- Salt to taste

INSTRUCTIONS:

1. Preheat oven to 400°F (200°C).
2. In a bowl, toss edamame with olive oil, chili powder, garlic powder, and salt.
3. Spread edamame in a single layer on a baking sheet.
4. Roast for 15-20 minutes, or until edamame are tender and slightly crispy.
5. Serve hot as a spicy and satisfying snack.

Caprese Skewers with Balsamic Glaze

INGREDIENTS:

- Cherry tomatoes
- Fresh mozzarella balls
- Fresh basil leaves
- Balsamic glaze
- Skewers

INSTRUCTIONS:

1. Thread cherry tomatoes, mozzarella balls, and basil leaves onto skewers.
2. Drizzle with balsamic glaze before serving.

Cucumber Roll-Ups with Herbed Cream Cheese

INGREDIENTS:

- 1 cucumber
- 1/2 cup cream cheese, softened

- 2 tablespoons chopped fresh herbs (such as dill, chives, or parsley)
- Salt and pepper to taste

INSTRUCTIONS:

1. Using a vegetable peeler, peel the cucumber into long, thin strips.
2. In a bowl, combine cream cheese, chopped herbs, salt, and pepper.
3. Spread a thin layer of the cream cheese mixture onto each cucumber strip.
4. Roll up the cucumber strips and secure with toothpicks.

Roasted Red Pepper and Feta Dip

INGREDIENTS:

- 1 jar (12 ounces) roasted red peppers, drained
- 4 ounces feta cheese
- 2 tablespoons olive oil

- 1 tablespoon lemon juice
- 1 clove garlic, minced
- Salt and pepper to taste

INSTRUCTIONS:

1. In a food processor, combine roasted red peppers, feta cheese, olive oil, lemon juice, garlic, salt, and pepper.
2. Blend until smooth.
3. Serve with pita chips or crudites for dipping.

Smoked Salmon Cucumber Bites

INGREDIENTS:

- 1 cucumber, sliced
- Smoked salmon
- Cream cheese
- Fresh dill

INSTRUCTIONS:

1. Top each cucumber slice with a small piece of smoked salmon.

2. Garnish with a small dollop of cream cheese and a sprig of fresh dill.

Stuffed Mini Bell Peppers

INGREDIENTS:

- Mini bell peppers
- Cream cheese
- Chopped fresh herbs (such as chives, parsley, or basil)
- Salt and pepper to taste

INSTRUCTIONS:

1. Cut the tops off the mini bell peppers and remove the seeds.

2. In a bowl, combine cream cheese, chopped herbs, salt, and pepper.

3. Spoon the cream cheese mixture into the peppers.

4. Serve as a delicious and colorful appetizer.

Greek Yogurt Ranch Dip with Veggies

INGREDIENTS:

- 1 cup Greek yogurt
- 1 tablespoon ranch seasoning mix
- Assorted raw vegetables (such as carrots, celery, and bell peppers) for dipping

INSTRUCTIONS:

1. In a bowl, combine Greek yogurt and ranch seasoning mix.
2. Stir until well combined.
3. Serve with assorted raw vegetables for dipping.

Almond Butter Energy Balls

INGREDIENTS:

- 1 cup rolled oats
- 1/2 cup almond butter
- 1/4 cup honey or maple syrup
- 1/4 cup chopped nuts

- 1/4 cup dried fruit (such as raisins or cranberries)
- 1/4 cup shredded coconut

INSTRUCTIONS:

1. In a bowl, combine rolled oats, almond butter, honey or maple syrup, chopped nuts, dried fruit, and shredded coconut.
2. Stir until well combined.
3. Roll the mixture into small balls.
4. Refrigerate for at least 30 minutes before serving.

CHAPTER 3: PASTA

Whole Wheat Spaghetti with Marinara Sauce

INGREDIENTS:

- Whole wheat spaghetti
- Marinara sauce
- Parmesan cheese (optional)

INSTRUCTIONS:

1. Cook whole wheat spaghetti according to package instructions.
2. Heat marinara sauce in a saucepan over medium heat.
3. Once spaghetti is cooked, drain and add to the saucepan with the marinara sauce.
4. Toss to combine and serve with grated Parmesan cheese if desired.

Pesto Pasta with Cherry Tomatoes and Arugula

INGREDIENTS:

- Pesto sauce
- Cherry tomatoes, halved
- Arugula
- Parmesan cheese (optional)

INSTRUCTIONS:

1. Cook pasta according to package instructions.
2. Drain pasta and return to the pot.
3. Add pesto sauce, cherry tomatoes, and arugula to the pot with the pasta.
4. Toss to combine and serve with grated Parmesan cheese if desired.

Zucchini Noodles with Lemon Garlic Shrimp

INGREDIENTS:

- Zucchini noodles

- Shrimp, peeled and deveined
- Lemon juice
- Garlic, minced
- Olive oil
- Salt and pepper

INSTRUCTIONS:

1. Heat olive oil in a large skillet over medium heat.
2. Add garlic and cook until fragrant, about 1 minute.
3. Add shrimp to the skillet and cook until pink and cooked through.
4. Add zucchini noodles to the skillet and cook until heated through.
5. Remove from heat and stir in lemon juice, salt, and pepper.
6. Serve hot.

One-Pot Pasta Primavera

INGREDIENTS:

- Whole grain pasta

- Mixed vegetables (such as bell peppers, broccoli, and carrots), chopped
- Vegetable broth
- Parmesan cheese (optional)

INSTRUCTIONS:

1. In a large pot, combine pasta, mixed vegetables, and vegetable broth.
2. Bring to a boil, then reduce heat and simmer until pasta is cooked and vegetables are tender, stirring occasionally.
3. Remove from heat and stir in Parmesan cheese if desired.
4. Serve hot.

Spicy Sausage and Kale Pasta

INGREDIENTS:

- Spicy sausage, sliced
- Kale, chopped
- Garlic, minced
- Crushed red pepper flakes

- Olive oil
- Parmesan cheese (optional)

INSTRUCTIONS:

1. Cook pasta according to package instructions.
2. In a large skillet, heat olive oil over medium heat.
3. Add garlic and cook until fragrant, about 1 minute.
4. Add sliced sausage to the skillet and cook until browned.
5. Add chopped kale and crushed red pepper flakes to the skillet and cook until kale is wilted.
6. Add cooked pasta to the skillet and toss to combine.
7. Serve hot with grated Parmesan cheese if desired.

Butternut Squash Ravioli with Sage Butter Sauce

INGREDIENTS:

- Butternut squash ravioli
- Butter
- Fresh sage leaves

- Parmesan cheese (optional)

INSTRUCTIONS:

1. Cook ravioli according to package instructions.
2. In a large skillet, melt butter over medium heat.
3. Add fresh sage leaves to the skillet and cook until crisp.
4. Remove sage leaves from the skillet and set aside.
5. Add cooked ravioli to the skillet and toss to coat in the sage butter sauce.
6. Serve hot with crispy sage leaves and grated Parmesan cheese if desired.

Creamy Mushroom and Spinach Pasta

INGREDIENTS:

- Mushrooms, sliced
- Spinach, chopped
- Garlic, minced
- Heavy cream

- Parmesan cheese
- Olive oil
- Salt and pepper

INSTRUCTIONS:

1. Cook pasta according to package instructions.
2. In a large skillet, heat olive oil over medium heat.
3. Add garlic and cook until fragrant, about 1 minute.
4. Add sliced mushrooms to the skillet and cook until browned.
5. Add chopped spinach to the skillet and cook until wilted.
6. Stir in heavy cream and Parmesan cheese, and cook until sauce is thickened.
7. Season with salt and pepper to taste.
8. Serve hot.

Eggplant and Tomato Pasta Bake

INGREDIENTS:

- Eggplant, diced
- Cherry tomatoes, halved
- Mozzarella cheese, shredded
- Parmesan cheese, grated
- Tomato sauce
- Olive oil
- Italian seasoning
- Salt and pepper

INSTRUCTIONS:

1. Preheat oven to 375°F (190°C).
2. In a large bowl, toss diced eggplant with olive oil, Italian seasoning, salt, and pepper.
3. Spread eggplant on a baking sheet and roast in the preheated oven for 20-25 minutes, or until tender.
4. In a large bowl, combine roasted eggplant, cherry tomatoes, tomato sauce, and cooked pasta.

5. Transfer mixture to a baking dish and top with shredded mozzarella cheese and grated Parmesan cheese.
6. Bake in the preheated oven for 20-25 minutes, or until cheese is melted and bubbly.
7. Serve hot.

Lentil Bolognese with Whole Grain Penne

INGREDIENTS:

- Whole grain penne
- Lentils, cooked
- Tomato sauce
- Onion, diced
- Carrot, diced
- Celery, diced
- Garlic, minced
- Olive oil
- Italian seasoning
- Salt and pepper

INSTRUCTIONS:

1. Cook pasta according to package instructions.
2. In a large skillet, heat olive oil over medium heat.
3. Add diced onion, carrot, celery, and garlic to the skillet and cook until softened.
4. Add cooked lentils, tomato sauce, Italian seasoning, salt, and pepper to the skillet.
5. Simmer for 15-20 minutes, stirring occasionally.
6. Serve lentil Bolognese over cooked whole grain penne.

Asian Peanut Noodle Salad

INGREDIENTS:

- Rice noodles
- Cucumber, julienned
- Carrot, julienned
- Bell pepper, julienned
- Green onions, sliced
- Cilantro, chopped
- Peanuts, chopped
- Sesame seeds
- Peanut butter

- Soy sauce
- Rice vinegar
- Honey
- Sriracha

INSTRUCTIONS:

1. Cook rice noodles according to package instructions.
2. In a large bowl, combine julienned cucumber, carrot, bell pepper, sliced green onions, and chopped cilantro.
3. In a small bowl, whisk together peanut butter, soy sauce, rice vinegar, honey, and sriracha to make the dressing.
4. Toss cooked rice noodles with vegetables and dressing.
5. Serve cold, garnished with chopped peanuts and sesame seeds.

CHAPTER 4: MEAT

Grilled Lemon Herb Chicken

INGREDIENTS:

- Chicken breasts
- Lemon juice
- Olive oil
- Garlic, minced
- Fresh herbs (such as rosemary, thyme, and oregano), chopped
- Salt and pepper

INSTRUCTIONS:

1. In a bowl, combine lemon juice, olive oil, minced garlic, chopped herbs, salt, and pepper.
2. Place chicken breasts in a resealable plastic bag and pour the marinade over them.
3. Seal the bag and refrigerate for at least 30 minutes, or overnight.
4. Preheat the grill to medium-high heat.

5. Grill chicken breasts for 6-7 minutes per side, or until cooked through.

6. Serve hot.

Turkey and Vegetable Stir-Fry

INGREDIENTS:

- Turkey breast, sliced
- Assorted vegetables (such as bell peppers, broccoli, and snap peas), sliced
- Soy sauce
- Garlic, minced
- Ginger, minced
- Olive oil
- Rice or noodles, cooked (optional)

INSTRUCTIONS:

1. In a large skillet or wok, heat olive oil over medium-high heat.

2. Add minced garlic and ginger to the skillet and cook until fragrant, about 1 minute.

3. Add sliced turkey breast to the skillet and cook until browned.

4. Add sliced vegetables to the skillet and cook until tender-crisp.

5. Stir in soy sauce and cook for an additional minute.

6. Serve stir-fry over cooked rice or noodles if desired.

Baked Salmon with Dill Sauce

INGREDIENTS:

- Salmon fillets
- Lemon juice
- Olive oil
- Garlic, minced
- Dill, chopped
- Salt and pepper

INSTRUCTIONS:

1. Preheat oven to 375°F (190°C).

2. In a bowl, combine lemon juice, olive oil, minced garlic, chopped dill, salt, and pepper.

3. Place salmon fillets on a baking sheet lined with parchment paper.
4. Brush salmon fillets with the lemon herb marinade.
5. Bake in the preheated oven for 12-15 minutes, or until salmon is cooked through.
6. Serve hot with dill sauce.

Moroccan Spiced Chicken Skewers

INGREDIENTS:

- Chicken thighs, cubed
- Moroccan spice blend
- Olive oil
- Lemon juice
- Salt and pepper

INSTRUCTIONS:

1. In a bowl, combine Moroccan spice blend, olive oil, lemon juice, salt, and pepper.
2. Add cubed chicken thighs to the bowl and toss to coat.

3. Cover and refrigerate for at least 30 minutes, or overnight.
4. Preheat the grill to medium-high heat.
5. Thread marinated chicken onto skewers.
6. Grill skewers for 5-6 minutes per side, or until chicken is cooked through.
7. Serve hot.

Beef and Broccoli Stir-Fry

INGREDIENTS:

- Beef sirloin, thinly sliced
- Broccoli florets
- Soy sauce
- Garlic, minced
- Ginger, minced
- Olive oil
- Rice or noodles, cooked (optional)

INSTRUCTIONS:

1. In a large skillet or wok, heat olive oil over medium-high heat.

2. Add minced garlic and ginger to the skillet and cook until fragrant, about 1 minute.
3. Add sliced beef sirloin to the skillet and cook until browned.
4. Add broccoli florets to the skillet and cook until tender-crisp.
5. Stir in soy sauce and cook for an additional minute.
6. Serve stir-fry over cooked rice or noodles if desired.

Lemon Garlic Herb Roast Chicken

INGREDIENTS:

- Whole chicken
- Lemon, sliced
- Garlic cloves, minced
- Fresh herbs (such as rosemary, thyme, and parsley), chopped
- Olive oil
- Salt and pepper

INSTRUCTIONS:

1. Preheat oven to 375°F (190°C).
2. Season whole chicken with salt, pepper, minced garlic, and chopped herbs.
3. Place lemon slices inside the cavity of the chicken.
4. Tie the legs together with kitchen twine.
5. Place the chicken on a roasting pan and drizzle with olive oil.
6. Roast in the preheated oven for 1-1.5 hours, or until the internal temperature reaches 165°F (74°C).
7. Let the chicken rest for 10 minutes before carving.
8. Serve hot.

Asian Turkey Lettuce Wraps

INGREDIENTS:

- Ground turkey
- Onion, diced
- Water chestnuts, diced
- Soy sauce
- Hoisin sauce
- Ginger, minced
- Garlic, minced

- Green onions, sliced
- Lettuce leaves

INSTRUCTIONS:

1. In a large skillet, cook ground turkey over medium heat until browned.

2. Add diced onion, water chestnuts, minced ginger, and minced garlic to the skillet and cook until onion is soft.

3. Stir in soy sauce and hoisin sauce, and cook for an additional minute.

4. Remove from heat and stir in sliced green onions.

5. Spoon the turkey mixture into lettuce leaves and serve.

Greek Lamb Meatballs with Tzatziki

INGREDIENTS:

- Ground lamb
- Onion, grated

- Garlic, minced
- Fresh mint, chopped
- Fresh parsley, chopped
- Salt and pepper
- Olive oil
- Tzatziki sauce (store-bought or homemade)

INSTRUCTIONS:

1. Preheat oven to 400°F (200°C).
2. In a bowl, combine ground lamb, grated onion, minced garlic, chopped mint, chopped parsley, salt, and pepper.
3. Shape the mixture into meatballs and place on a baking sheet lined with parchment paper.
4. Drizzle meatballs with olive oil and bake in the preheated oven for 15-20 minutes, or until cooked through.
5. Serve meatballs with tzatziki sauce.

CHAPTER 5: FISH

Baked Cod with Lemon and Herbs

INGREDIENTS:

- Cod fillets
- Lemon juice
- Olive oil
- Garlic, minced
- Fresh herbs (such as parsley and thyme), chopped
- Salt and pepper

INSTRUCTIONS:

1. Preheat oven to 400°F (200°C).
2. Place cod fillets on a baking sheet lined with parchment paper.
3. In a bowl, combine lemon juice, olive oil, minced garlic, chopped herbs, salt, and pepper.
4. Pour the lemon herb mixture over the cod fillets.

5. Bake in the preheated oven for 15-20 minutes, or until fish is cooked through and flakes easily with a fork.

6. Serve hot.

Grilled Mahi-Mahi with Pineapple Salsa

INGREDIENTS:

- Mahi-mahi fillets
- Olive oil
- Lime juice
- Garlic powder
- Paprika
- Salt and pepper
- Pineapple salsa (store-bought or homemade)

INSTRUCTIONS:

1. Preheat the grill to medium-high heat.

2. Brush mahi-mahi fillets with olive oil and sprinkle with lime juice, garlic powder, paprika, salt, and pepper.

3. Grill mahi-mahi fillets for 3-4 minutes per side, or until fish is cooked through and flakes easily with a fork.
4. Serve hot with pineapple salsa.

Pan-Seared Trout with Almond Brown Butter

INGREDIENTS:

- Trout fillets
- Flour
- Butter
- Slivered almonds
- Lemon juice
- Fresh parsley, chopped
- Salt and pepper

INSTRUCTIONS:

1. Season trout fillets with salt and pepper, and dredge in flour.
2. In a large skillet, melt butter over medium heat.

3. Add slivered almonds to the skillet and cook until lightly toasted.

4. Remove almonds from the skillet and set aside.

5. Increase heat to medium-high and add trout fillets to the skillet.

6. Cook trout fillets for 3-4 minutes per side, or until fish is cooked through and flakes easily with a fork.

7. Remove trout fillets from the skillet and keep warm.

8. Add lemon juice and chopped parsley to the skillet and cook until butter is browned.

9. Pour almond brown butter over trout fillets and serve hot.

Teriyaki Salmon with Sesame Seeds

INGREDIENTS:

- Salmon fillets
- Teriyaki sauce
- Sesame seeds
- Green onions, sliced
- Cooked rice, for serving

INSTRUCTIONS:

1. Preheat oven to 400°F (200°C).
2. Place salmon fillets on a baking sheet lined with parchment paper.
3. Brush salmon fillets with teriyaki sauce and sprinkle with sesame seeds.
4. Bake in the preheated oven for 12-15 minutes, or until salmon is cooked through and flakes easily with a fork.
5. Serve hot over cooked rice, and garnish with sliced green onions.

Coconut Curry Shrimp

INGREDIENTS:

- Shrimp, peeled and deveined
- Coconut milk
- Red curry paste
- Fish sauce
- Brown sugar
- Lime juice

- Fresh cilantro, chopped
- Cooked rice, for serving

INSTRUCTIONS:

1. In a large skillet, combine coconut milk, red curry paste, fish sauce, brown sugar, and lime juice.
2. Bring to a simmer over medium heat.
3. Add shrimp to the skillet and cook for 5-6 minutes, or until shrimp are pink and cooked through.
4. Stir in chopped cilantro.
5. Serve hot over cooked rice.

Lemon Dill Baked Halibut

INGREDIENTS:

- Halibut fillets
- Lemon juice
- Olive oil
- Garlic, minced
- Fresh dill, chopped
- Salt and pepper

INSTRUCTIONS:

1. Preheat oven to 400°F (200°C).
2. Place halibut fillets on a baking sheet lined with parchment paper.
3. In a bowl, combine lemon juice, olive oil, minced garlic, chopped dill, salt, and pepper.
4. Pour the lemon dill mixture over the halibut fillets.
5. Bake in the preheated oven for 15-20 minutes, or until fish is cooked through and flakes easily with a fork.
6. Serve hot.

Tuna Nicoise Salad

INGREDIENTS:

- Tuna steaks
- Mixed salad greens
- Cherry tomatoes, halved
- Hard-boiled eggs, sliced
- Green beans blanched
- Kalamata olives

- Red onion, thinly sliced
- Lemon juice
- Olive oil
- Dijon mustard
- Salt and pepper

INSTRUCTIONS:

1. Season tuna steaks with salt and pepper.
2. Heat olive oil in a skillet over medium-high heat.
3. Sear tuna steaks for 1-2 minutes per side, or until desired doneness.
4. In a small bowl, whisk together lemon juice, olive oil, Dijon mustard, salt, and pepper to make the dressing.
5. In a large bowl, combine mixed salad greens, halved cherry tomatoes, sliced hard-boiled eggs, blanched green beans, Kalamata olives, and thinly sliced red onion.
6. Toss salad with dressing.
7. Serve tuna steaks on top of the salad.

Blackened Catfish Tacos

INGREDIENTS:

- Catfish fillets
- Blackening seasoning
- Corn tortillas
- Coleslaw mix
- Avocado, sliced
- Lime wedges

INSTRUCTIONS:

1. Season catfish fillets with blackening seasoning.
2. Heat olive oil in a skillet over medium-high heat.
3. Cook catfish fillets for 3-4 minutes per side, or until fish is cooked through and flakes easily with a fork.
4. Heat corn tortillas in a dry skillet until warmed.
5. Assemble tacos with coleslaw mix, sliced avocado, and cooked catfish.
6. Serve with lime wedges.

Mediterranean Stuffed Squid

INGREDIENTS:

- Squid tubes
- Olive oil
- Onion, diced
- Garlic, minced
- Tomato, diced
- Kalamata olives, chopped
- Feta cheese, crumbled
- Fresh parsley, chopped
- Lemon juice
- Salt and pepper

INSTRUCTIONS:

1. Preheat oven to 375°F (190°C).
2. In a skillet, heat olive oil over medium heat.
3. Add diced onion and minced garlic to the skillet and cook until softened.
4. Add diced tomato, chopped Kalamata olives, crumbled feta cheese, chopped parsley, lemon juice, salt, and pepper to the skillet.

5. Stir to combine and remove from heat.

6. Stuff squid tubes with the mixture and secure them with toothpicks.

7. Place stuffed squid tubes on a baking dish and drizzle with olive oil.

8. Bake in the preheated oven for 25-30 minutes, or until squid is cooked through.

9. Serve hot.

Salmon Burgers with Avocado Aioli

INGREDIENTS:

- Salmon fillets
- Bread crumbs
- Egg
- Dijon mustard
- Worcestershire sauce
- Salt and pepper
- Burger buns
- Avocado, mashed
- Mayonnaise

- Lemon juice
- Garlic, minced
- Lettuce and tomato, for serving

INSTRUCTIONS:

1. In a food processor, pulse salmon fillets until finely chopped.
2. In a bowl, combine chopped salmon, bread crumbs, egg, Dijon mustard, Worcestershire sauce, salt, and pepper.
3. Form the mixture into patties.
4. Heat olive oil in a skillet over medium heat.
5. Cook salmon patties for 3-4 minutes per side, or until cooked through.
6. In a small bowl, combine mashed avocado, mayonnaise, lemon juice, minced garlic, salt, and pepper to make the avocado aioli.
7. Serve salmon burgers on burger buns with avocado aioli, lettuce, and tomato.

CHAPTER 6: SALADS

Classic Caesar Salad

INGREDIENTS:

- Romaine lettuce, chopped
- Caesar dressing
- Parmesan cheese, grated
- Croutons

INSTRUCTIONS:

1. In a large bowl, combine chopped romaine lettuce and Caesar dressing.
2. Toss to coat the lettuce evenly.
3. Add grated Parmesan cheese and croutons.
4. Toss again to combine.
5. Serve immediately.

Greek Salad with Feta and Olives

INGREDIENTS:

- Cucumber, diced
- Tomatoes, diced
- Red onion, thinly sliced
- Kalamata olives
- Feta cheese, crumbled
- Olive oil
- Red wine vinegar
- Dried oregano
- Salt and pepper

INSTRUCTIONS:

1. In a large bowl, combine diced cucumber, diced tomatoes, thinly sliced red onion, Kalamata olives, and crumbled feta cheese.
2. In a small bowl, whisk together olive oil, red wine vinegar, dried oregano, salt, and pepper to make the dressing.

3. Pour the dressing over the salad and toss to combine.
4. Serve immediately.

Spinach Strawberry Salad with Balsamic Glaze

INGREDIENTS:

- Baby spinach
- Strawberries, sliced
- Red onion, thinly sliced
- Candied pecans
- Balsamic glaze

INSTRUCTIONS:

1. In a large bowl, combine baby spinach, sliced strawberries, thinly sliced red onion, and candied pecans.
2. Drizzle with balsamic glaze.
3. Toss to combine.
4. Serve immediately.

Waldorf Salad with Grilled Chicken

INGREDIENTS:

- Grilled chicken breast, sliced
- Apple diced
- Celery, diced
- Grapes, halved
- Walnuts, chopped
- Greek yogurt
- Lemon juice
- Honey
- Salt and pepper
- Lettuce leaves

INSTRUCTIONS:

1. In a large bowl, combine sliced grilled chicken breast, diced apple, diced celery, halved grapes, and chopped walnuts.

2. In a small bowl, whisk together Greek yogurt, lemon juice, honey, salt, and pepper to make the dressing.

3. Pour the dressing over the salad and toss to combine.
4. Serve on lettuce leaves.

Cobb Salad with Creamy Avocado Dressing

INGREDIENTS:

- Mixed salad greens
- Grilled chicken breast, diced
- Bacon, cooked and crumbled
- Hard-boiled eggs, sliced
- Avocado, diced
- Cherry tomatoes, halved
- Blue cheese, crumbled
- Creamy avocado dressing

INSTRUCTIONS:

1. Arrange mixed salad greens on a plate.
2. Top with diced grilled chicken breast, crumbled bacon, sliced hard-boiled eggs, diced avocado, halved cherry tomatoes, and crumbled blue cheese.
3. Drizzle with creamy avocado dressing.

4. Serve immediately.

Caprese Salad with Basil Pesto

INGREDIENTS:

- Fresh mozzarella cheese, sliced
- Tomatoes, sliced
- Fresh basil leaves
- Basil pesto
- Balsamic glaze

INSTRUCTIONS:

1. Arrange slices of fresh mozzarella cheese and tomatoes on a plate.
2. Top with fresh basil leaves.
3. Drizzle with basil pesto and balsamic glaze.
4. Serve immediately.

Asian Sesame Chicken Salad

INGREDIENTS:

- Mixed salad greens

- Grilled chicken breast, sliced
- Red bell pepper, julienned
- Carrots, julienned
- Edamame
- Green onions, sliced
- Sesame seeds
- Asian sesame dressing

INSTRUCTIONS:

1. Arrange mixed salad greens on a plate.
2. Top with sliced grilled chicken breast, julienned red bell pepper, julienned carrots, edamame, sliced green onions, and sesame seeds.
3. Drizzle with Asian sesame dressing.
4. Serve immediately.

Quinoa and Kale Salad with Lemon Vinaigrette

INGREDIENTS:

- Cooked quinoa
- Kale, chopped

- Cherry tomatoes, halved
- Cucumber, diced
- Red onion, thinly sliced
- Feta cheese, crumbled
- Lemon vinaigrette

INSTRUCTIONS:

1. In a large bowl, combine cooked quinoa, chopped kale, halved cherry tomatoes, diced cucumber, thinly sliced red onion, and crumbled feta cheese.
2. Drizzle with lemon vinaigrette.
3. Toss to combine.
4. Serve immediately.

Mexican Street Corn Salad

INGREDIENTS:

- Corn kernels, grilled
- Red onion, finely chopped
- Jalapeno, finely chopped
- Fresh cilantro, chopped
- Cotija cheese, crumbled

- Lime juice
- Mayonnaise
- Chili powder
- Salt and pepper

INSTRUCTIONS:

1. In a large bowl, combine grilled corn kernels, finely chopped red onion, finely chopped jalapeno, chopped fresh cilantro, and crumbled Cotija cheese.
2. In a small bowl, whisk together lime juice, mayonnaise, chili powder, salt, and pepper to make the dressing.
3. Pour the dressing over the salad and toss to combine.
4. Serve immediately.

Warm Lentil Salad with Roasted Vegetables

INGREDIENTS:

- Lentils, cooked
- Sweet potatoes, diced

- Red bell pepper, diced
- Red onion, sliced
- Olive oil
- Balsamic vinegar
- Dijon mustard
- Honey
- Salt and pepper
- Fresh parsley, chopped

INSTRUCTIONS:

1. Preheat oven to 400°F (200°C).
2. In a large bowl, combine diced sweet potatoes, diced red bell pepper, and sliced red onion.
3. Drizzle with olive oil and season with salt and pepper.
4. Spread the vegetables in a single layer on a baking sheet lined with parchment paper.
5. Roast in the preheated oven for 25-30 minutes, or until vegetables are tender and caramelized.
6. In a small bowl, whisk together balsamic vinegar, Dijon mustard, honey, salt, and pepper to make the dressing.

7. In a large bowl, combine cooked lentils, roasted vegetables, and chopped fresh parsley.

8. Pour the dressing over the salad and toss to combine.

9. Serve warm.

CHAPTER 7: SOUP & STEW

Lentil and Vegetable Stew

INGREDIENTS:

- Cooked lentils
- Mixed vegetables (such as carrots, celery, and bell peppers), diced
- Onion, diced
- Garlic, minced
- Vegetable broth
- Tomato paste
- Italian seasoning
- Salt and pepper
- Olive oil

INSTRUCTIONS:

1. In a large pot, heat olive oil over medium heat.
2. Add diced onion and minced garlic to the pot and cook until softened.
3. Add diced mixed vegetables to the pot and cook for a few minutes.

4. Stir in cooked lentils, vegetable broth, tomato paste, Italian seasoning, salt, and pepper.

5. Bring the stew to a simmer and cook for about 20-30 minutes, or until the vegetables are tender.

6. Serve hot.

Tomato Basil Soup with Parmesan Crisps

INGREDIENTS:

- Canned tomatoes
- Onion, diced
- Garlic, minced
- Vegetable broth
- Fresh basil leaves, chopped
- Heavy cream
- Parmesan cheese
- Olive oil
- Salt and pepper

INSTRUCTIONS:

1. In a large pot, heat olive oil over medium heat.

2. Add diced onion and minced garlic to the pot and cook until softened.

3. Add canned tomatoes, vegetable broth, and chopped fresh basil leaves to the pot.

4. Season with salt and pepper.

5. Bring the soup to a simmer and cook for about 15-20 minutes.

6. Use an immersion blender to blend the soup until smooth.

7. Stir in heavy cream.

8. To make Parmesan crisps, preheat oven to 400°F (200°C).

9. Line a baking sheet with parchment paper and place small mounds of grated Parmesan cheese on the paper.

10. Bake in the preheated oven for 5-7 minutes, or until the cheese is melted and golden brown.

11. Serve the soup hot with Parmesan crisps on top.

Chicken and Rice Soup

INGREDIENTS:

- Chicken breast, cooked and shredded
- Onion, diced
- Carrots, diced
- Celery, diced
- Garlic, minced
- Chicken broth
- Cooked rice
- Fresh thyme leaves
- Salt and pepper
- Olive oil

INSTRUCTIONS:

1. In a large pot, heat olive oil over medium heat.
2. Add diced onion, carrots, celery, and minced garlic to the pot and cook until softened.
3. Add shredded cooked chicken breast, chicken broth, cooked rice, fresh thyme leaves, salt, and pepper to the pot.

4. Bring the soup to a simmer and cook for about 10-15 minutes, or until the vegetables are tender.

5. Serve hot.

Butternut Squash and Apple Soup

INGREDIENTS:

- Butternut squash, peeled, seeded, and diced
- Apple, peeled, cored, and diced
- Onion, diced
- Garlic, minced
- Vegetable broth
- Coconut milk
- Curry powder
- Ground cinnamon
- Salt and pepper
- Olive oil

INSTRUCTIONS:

1. In a large pot, heat olive oil over medium heat.

2. Add diced onion and minced garlic to the pot and cook until softened.

3. Add diced butternut squash, diced apple, vegetable broth, curry powder, ground cinnamon, salt, and pepper to the pot.

4. Bring the soup to a simmer and cook for about 20-25 minutes, or until the squash and apple are tender.

5. Use an immersion blender to blend the soup until smooth.

6. Stir in coconut milk.

7. Serve hot.

Thai Coconut Curry Soup

INGREDIENTS:

- Red curry paste
- Coconut milk
- Vegetable broth
- Onion, thinly sliced
- Red bell pepper, thinly sliced
- Carrots, thinly sliced
- Mushrooms, sliced

- Cooked chicken, shredded
- Fresh cilantro, chopped
- Lime juice
- Salt and pepper
- Olive oil

INSTRUCTIONS:

1. In a large pot, heat olive oil over medium heat.
2. Add red curry paste to the pot and cook for a minute.
3. Add thinly sliced onion, red bell pepper, carrots, and mushrooms to the pot and cook until softened.
4. Stir in coconut milk and vegetable broth.
5. Add shredded cooked chicken to the pot.
6. Bring the soup to a simmer and cook for about 10-15 minutes.
7. Stir in chopped fresh cilantro and lime juice.
8. Season with salt and pepper.
9. Serve hot.

Minestrone Soup with White Beans and Pasta

INGREDIENTS:

- Onion, diced
- Carrots, diced
- Celery, diced
- Garlic, minced
- Vegetable broth
- Canned diced tomatoes
- Cannellini beans drained and rinsed
- Small pasta (such as ditalini or small shells)
- Fresh basil leaves, chopped
- Fresh parsley, chopped
- Grated Parmesan cheese
- Olive oil
- Salt and pepper

INSTRUCTIONS:

1. In a large pot, heat olive oil over medium heat.

2. Add diced onion, carrots, celery, and minced garlic to the pot and cook until softened.

3. Add vegetable broth, canned diced tomatoes, and drained and rinsed cannellini beans to the pot.

4. Bring the soup to a simmer and cook for about 10-15 minutes.

5. Add small pasta to the pot and cook according to package instructions.

6. Stir in chopped fresh basil leaves and parsley.

7. Serve hot with grated Parmesan cheese on top.

Spicy Black Bean Soup

INGREDIENTS:

- Black beans, cooked
- Onion, diced
- Red bell pepper, diced
- Jalapeno pepper, diced
- Garlic, minced
- Vegetable broth
- Canned diced tomatoes
- Ground cumin

- Chili powder
- Cayenne pepper
- Salt and pepper
- Olive oil

INSTRUCTIONS:

1. In a large pot, heat olive oil over medium heat.
2. Add diced onion, red bell pepper, jalapeno pepper, and minced garlic to the pot and cook until softened.
3. Add cooked black beans, vegetable broth, canned diced tomatoes, ground cumin, chili powder, cayenne pepper, salt, and pepper to the pot.
4. Bring the soup to a simmer and cook for about 15-20 minutes.
5. Use an immersion blender to blend a portion of the soup until smooth.
6. Serve hot.

Moroccan Chickpea Stew

INGREDIENTS:

- Onion, diced

- Carrots, diced
- Celery, diced
- Garlic, minced
- Vegetable broth
- Canned chickpeas, drained and rinsed
- Canned diced tomatoes
- Ground cumin
- Ground coriander
- Ground cinnamon
- Ground ginger
- Paprika
- Salt and pepper
- Olive oil

INSTRUCTIONS:

1. In a large pot, heat olive oil over medium heat.
2. Add diced onion, carrots, celery, and minced garlic to the pot and cook until softened.
3. Add vegetable broth, drained and rinsed chickpeas, canned diced tomatoes, ground cumin, ground coriander, ground cinnamon, ground ginger, paprika, salt, and pepper to the pot.

4. Bring the stew to a simmer and cook for about 20-25 minutes.

5. Serve hot.

Creamy Mushroom Soup

INGREDIENTS:

- Assorted mushrooms, sliced
- Onion, diced
- Garlic, minced
- Vegetable broth
- Heavy cream
- Fresh thyme leaves
- Salt and pepper
- Olive oil

INSTRUCTIONS:

1. In a large pot, heat olive oil over medium heat.
2. Add sliced assorted mushrooms to the pot and cook until softened.
3. Add diced onion and minced garlic to the pot and cook until softened.

4. Stir in vegetable broth and bring the soup to a simmer.

5. Use an immersion blender to blend a portion of the soup until smooth.

6. Stir in heavy cream and fresh thyme leaves.

7. Season with salt and pepper.

8. Serve hot.

Sweet Potato and Kale Soup

INGREDIENTS:

- Sweet potatoes, peeled and diced
- Onion, diced
- Garlic, minced
- Vegetable broth
- Coconut milk
- Kale, chopped
- Ground cumin
- Ground coriander
- Ground cinnamon
- Ground nutmeg
- Salt and pepper

- Olive oil

INSTRUCTIONS:

1. In a large pot, heat olive oil over medium heat.
2. Add diced onion and minced garlic to the pot and cook until softened.
3. Add diced sweet potatoes to the pot and cook for a few minutes.
4. Stir in vegetable broth, coconut milk, ground cumin, ground coriander, ground cinnamon, ground nutmeg, salt, and pepper.
5. Bring the soup to a simmer and cook for about 20-25 minutes, or until the sweet potatoes are tender.
6. Use an immersion blender to blend a portion of the soup until smooth.
7. Stir in chopped kale and cook for another 5 minutes, or until the kale is wilted.
8. Serve hot.

CHAPTER 8: DESSERTS

Dark Chocolate Covered Strawberries

INGREDIENTS:

- Fresh strawberries
- Dark chocolate chips
- Coconut oil

INSTRUCTIONS:

1. Wash and dry the strawberries thoroughly.
2. In a microwave-safe bowl, melt the dark chocolate chips with coconut oil in 30-second intervals, stirring in between, until smooth.
3. Dip each strawberry into the melted chocolate, coating it halfway.
4. Place the dipped strawberries on a parchment-lined baking sheet.
5. Refrigerate for about 30 minutes, or until the chocolate is set.
6. Serve and enjoy!

Baked Apples with Cinnamon and Honey

INGREDIENTS:

- Apples, cored and sliced
- Cinnamon
- Honey
- Oats (optional)
- Chopped nuts (optional)

INSTRUCTIONS:

1. Preheat the oven to 350°F (175°C).
2. Place the sliced apples in a baking dish.
3. Sprinkle cinnamon over the apples and drizzle with honey.
4. Optional: Sprinkle oats and chopped nuts over the apples for added texture.
5. Bake for about 20-25 minutes, or until the apples are tender.
6. Serve warm.

Greek Yogurt Popsicles with Fresh Berries

INGREDIENTS:

- Greek yogurt
- Fresh berries (such as strawberries, blueberries, and raspberries)
- Honey (optional)

INSTRUCTIONS:

1. In a bowl, mix the Greek yogurt with honey, if desired.
2. Layer the yogurt and fresh berries in popsicle molds.
3. Insert popsicle sticks into the molds.
4. Freeze for at least 4 hours, or until solid.
5. Remove the popsicles from the molds and enjoy!

Coconut Chia Seed Pudding

INGREDIENTS:

- Coconut milk
- Chia seeds

- Maple syrup or honey
- Vanilla extract
- Fresh berries (optional)

INSTRUCTIONS:

1. In a bowl, mix coconut milk, chia seeds, maple syrup or honey, and vanilla extract.
2. Stir well to combine.
3. Cover and refrigerate overnight, or for at least 4 hours, to allow the chia seeds to thicken.
4. Serve chilled, topped with fresh berries if desired.

Banana Almond Butter Bites

INGREDIENTS:

- Bananas, peeled and sliced
- Almond butter
- Dark chocolate chips (optional)
- Chopped nuts (optional)

INSTRUCTIONS:

1. Spread almond butter on banana slices.
2. Optional: Melt dark chocolate chips and drizzle over the almond butter.
3. Optional: Sprinkle chopped nuts over the almond butter.
4. Freeze for about 1 hour, or until firm.
5. Serve as a healthy and delicious treat.

Berry Sorbet

INGREDIENTS:

- Frozen mixed berries
- Honey or maple syrup (optional)
- Lemon juice

INSTRUCTIONS:

1. In a blender or food processor, blend frozen mixed berries until smooth.
2. Add honey or maple syrup, if desired, and lemon juice to taste.
3. Blend again until well combined.
4. Serve immediately as a refreshing sorbet.

Pumpkin Pie Bites

INGREDIENTS:

- Pumpkin puree
- Maple syrup or honey
- Pumpkin pie spice
- Graham cracker crumbs
- Cream cheese (optional)
- Whipped cream (optional)

INSTRUCTIONS:

1. In a bowl, mix pumpkin puree, maple syrup or honey, and pumpkin pie spice.
2. Roll the mixture into bite-sized balls.
3. Roll the balls in graham cracker crumbs to coat.
4. Optional: Serve with a dollop of cream cheese or whipped cream on top.

Chocolate Avocado Mousse

INGREDIENTS:

- Ripe avocados

- Cocoa powder
- Maple syrup or honey
- Vanilla extract
- Almond milk (optional)

INSTRUCTIONS:

1. In a blender or food processor, blend ripe avocados until smooth.
2. Add cocoa powder, maple syrup or honey, and vanilla extract to taste.
3. Optional: Add a splash of almond milk for a creamier texture.
4. Blend again until well combined.
5. Serve chilled.

Lemon Blueberry Yogurt Cake

INGREDIENTS:

- Greek yogurt
- Lemon zest
- Lemon juice
- Blueberries

- Flour
- Baking powder
- Baking soda
- Salt
- Sugar
- Eggs
- Olive oil

INSTRUCTIONS:

1. In a bowl, mix Greek yogurt, lemon zest, and lemon juice.
2. In another bowl, whisk together flour, baking powder, baking soda, and salt.
3. In a separate bowl, beat sugar, eggs, and olive oil until light and fluffy.
4. Gradually add the flour mixture to the egg mixture, alternating with the yogurt mixture.
5. Gently fold in blueberries.
6. Pour the batter into a greased loaf pan.
7. Bake at 350°F (175°C) for about 50-60 minutes, or until a toothpick inserted into the center comes out clean.

8. Let cool before slicing and serving.

Oatmeal Raisin Energy Balls

INGREDIENTS:

- Rolled oats
- Raisins
- Almond butter
- Honey
- Vanilla extract
- Ground cinnamon
- Chia seeds (optional)

INSTRUCTIONS:

1. In a food processor, blend rolled oats until they form a fine flour-like consistency.
2. Add raisins, almond butter, honey, vanilla extract, ground cinnamon, and chia seeds, if using.
3. Blend until the mixture comes together and can be formed into balls.
4. Roll the mixture into bite-sized balls.
5. Refrigerate for at least 30 minutes, or until firm.

6. Serve as a healthy and energy-boosting snack.

CHAPTER 9: SMOOTHIES & BEVERAGES

Green Detox Smoothie

INGREDIENTS:

- Spinach
- Kale
- Cucumber
- Celery
- Green apple
- Lemon juice
- Ginger
- Water or coconut water
- Ice cubes

INSTRUCTIONS:

1. In a blender, combine spinach, kale, cucumber, celery, green apple, lemon juice, ginger, water or coconut water, and ice cubes.
2. Blend until smooth.
3. Serve immediately.

Berry Blast Smoothie with Spinach

INGREDIENTS:

- Mixed berries (such as strawberries, blueberries, and raspberries)
- Spinach
- Greek yogurt
- Almond milk
- Honey or maple syrup (optional)
- Ice cubes

INSTRUCTIONS:

1. In a blender, combine mixed berries, spinach, Greek yogurt, almond milk, honey or maple syrup, and ice cubes.
2. Blend until smooth.
3. Serve immediately.

Mango Coconut Water Smoothie

Ingredients:

- Mango
- Coconut water
- Banana
- Lime juice
- Coconut flakes (optional)
- Ice cubes

Instructions:

1. In a blender, combine mango, coconut water, banana, lime juice, coconut flakes, and ice cubes.
2. Blend until smooth.
3. Serve immediately.

Peanut Butter Banana Protein Smoothie

INGREDIENTS:

- Banana
- Peanut butter

- Protein powder
- Almond milk
- Honey or maple syrup (optional)
- Ice cubes

INSTRUCTIONS:

1. In a blender, combine banana, peanut butter, protein powder, almond milk, honey or maple syrup, and ice cubes.
2. Blend until smooth.
3. Serve immediately.

Iced Turmeric Latte

INGREDIENTS:

- Turmeric powder
- Cinnamon
- Ginger
- Honey
- Almond milk
- Espresso or strong coffee
- Ice cubes

INSTRUCTIONS:

1. In a small saucepan, combine turmeric powder, cinnamon, ginger, honey, and almond milk.
2. Heat over medium heat until warm, stirring occasionally.
3. Remove from heat and let cool.
4. In a glass, combine the turmeric mixture with espresso or strong coffee and ice cubes.
5. Stir well and serve.

Cucumber Mint Cooler

INGREDIENTS:

- Cucumber
- Mint leaves
- Lime juice
- Honey or agave syrup
- Water
- Ice cubes

INSTRUCTIONS:

1. In a blender, combine cucumber, mint leaves, lime juice, honey or agave syrup, water, and ice cubes.
2. Blend until smooth.
3. Serve immediately.

Matcha Green Tea Smoothie

INGREDIENTS:

- Matcha green tea powder
- Spinach
- Banana
- Almond milk
- Honey or maple syrup (optional)
- Ice cubes

INSTRUCTIONS:

1. In a blender, combine matcha green tea powder, spinach, banana, almond milk, honey or maple syrup, and ice cubes.

2. Blend until smooth.

3. Serve immediately.

Watermelon Lime Slushie

INGREDIENTS:

- Watermelon
- Lime juice
- Mint leaves
- Water
- Ice cubes

INSTRUCTIONS:

1. In a blender, combine watermelon, lime juice, mint leaves, water, and ice cubes.

2. Blend until smooth.

3. Serve immediately.

Golden Milk Latte

INGREDIENTS:

- Turmeric powder
- Cinnamon

- Ginger
- Black pepper
- Honey
- Almond milk
- Vanilla extract
- Ice cubes

INSTRUCTIONS:

1. In a small saucepan, combine turmeric powder, cinnamon, ginger, black pepper, honey, almond milk, and vanilla extract.
2. Heat over medium heat until warm, stirring occasionally.
3. Remove from heat and let cool.
4. In a glass, combine the turmeric mixture with ice cubes.
5. Stir well and serve.

Blueberry Kombucha

INGREDIENTS:

- Blueberries
- Kombucha

- Lemon juice
- Honey or agave syrup (optional)
- Ice cubes

INSTRUCTIONS:

1. In a blender, combine blueberries, kombucha, lemon juice, honey or agave syrup, and ice cubes.
2. Blend until smooth.
3. Serve immediately.

MEAL PLAN

Day 1:

- **Breakfast:** Greek Yogurt Parfait with Berries (Chapter 1, Recipe 2)
- **Lunch:** Lentil Bolognese with Whole Grain Penne (Chapter 3, Recipe 9)
- **Dinner:** Grilled Lemon Herb Chicken (Chapter 4, Recipe 1) with a side of Spinach Strawberry Salad with Balsamic Glaze (Chapter 6, Recipe 3)
- **Snack:** Banana Almond Butter Bites (Chapter 8, Recipe 5)

Day 2:

- **Breakfast:** Blueberry Banana Smoothie (Chapter 1, Recipe 6)
- **Lunch:** Butternut Squash and Apple Soup (Chapter 7, Recipe 4)
- **Dinner:** Moroccan Spiced Chicken Skewers (Chapter 4, Recipe 4) with a side of Mexican Street Corn Salad (Chapter 6, Recipe 9)
- **Snack:** Coconut Chia Seed Pudding (Chapter 8, Recipe 4)

Day 3:

- **Breakfast:** Avocado Toast with Poached Egg (Chapter 1, Recipe 5)
- **Lunch:** Creamy Mushroom and Spinach Pasta (Chapter 3, Recipe 7)
- **Dinner:** Baked Cod with Lemon and Herbs (Chapter 5, Recipe 1) served with a side of Warm Lentil Salad with Roasted Vegetables (Chapter 6, Recipe 10)
- **Snack:** Dark Chocolate Covered Strawberries (Chapter 8, Recipe 1)

Day 4:

- **Breakfast:** Chia Seed Pudding with Almond Milk (Chapter 1, Recipe 4)
- **Lunch:** Asian Peanut Noodle Salad (Chapter 3, Recipe 10)
- **Dinner:** Turkey and Vegetable Stir-Fry (Chapter 4, Recipe 2)
- **Snack:** Hummus with Crudites (Chapter 2, Recipe 2)

Day 5:

- **Breakfast:** Whole Grain Pancakes with Maple Syrup (Chapter 1, Recipe 7)
- **Lunch:** Tomato Basil Soup with Parmesan Crisps (Chapter 7, Recipe 2)
- **Dinner:** Lemon Garlic Herb Roast Chicken (Chapter 4, Recipe 6) with a side of Spinach Strawberry Salad with Balsamic Glaze (Chapter 6, Recipe 3)
- **Snack:** Greek Yogurt Ranch Dip with Veggies (Chapter 2, Recipe 9)

Day 6:

- **Breakfast:** Quinoa Breakfast Bowl with Nuts and Seeds (Chapter 1, Recipe 9)
- **Lunch:** Lentil and Vegetable Stew (Chapter 6, Recipe 1)
- **Dinner:** Beef and Broccoli Stir-Fry (Chapter 4, Recipe 6)
- **Snack:** Guacamole with Baked Tortilla Chips (Chapter 2, Recipe 1)

Day 7:

- **Breakfast:** Sweet Potato Hash with Turkey Sausage (Chapter 1, Recipe 10)

- **Lunch:** Chicken and Rice Soup (Chapter 7, Recipe 3)
- **Dinner:** Mexican Street Corn Salad (Chapter 6, Recipe 9)
- **Snack:** Almond Butter Energy Balls (Chapter 2, Recipe 10)

Day 8:
- **Breakfast:** Berry Sorbet (Chapter 8, Recipe 6)
- **Lunch:** Spicy Black Bean Soup (Chapter 7, Recipe 7)
- **Dinner:** Grilled Mahi-Mahi with Pineapple Salsa (Chapter 5, Recipe 2) served with a side of Greek Salad with Feta and Olives (Chapter 6, Recipe 2)
- **Snack:** Lemon Blueberry Yogurt Cake (Chapter 8, Recipe 9)

Day 9:
- **Breakfast:** Pumpkin Pie Bites (Chapter 8, Recipe 7)
- **Lunch:** Creamy Mushroom Soup (Chapter 7, Recipe 9)
- **Dinner:** Moroccan Chickpea Stew (Chapter 6, Recipe 8)

- **Snack:** Stuffed Mini Bell Peppers (Chapter 2, Recipe 8)

Day 10:

- **Breakfast:** Chocolate Avocado Mousse (Chapter 8, Recipe 8)
- **Lunch:** Butternut Squash and Apple Soup (Chapter 7, Recipe 4)
- **Dinner:** Lemon Dill Baked Halibut (Chapter 5, Recipe 6) with a side of Greek Salad with Feta and Olives (Chapter 7, Recipe 2)
- **Snack:** Greek Yogurt Popsicles with Fresh Berries (Chapter 6, Recipe 3)

Day 11:

- **Breakfast:** Oatmeal Raisin Energy Balls (Chapter 8, Recipe 10)
- **Lunch:** Thai Coconut Curry Soup (Chapter 7, Recipe 5)
- **Dinner:** Asian Turkey Lettuce Wraps (Chapter 4, Recipe 8)
- **Snack:** Peanut Butter Banana Protein Smoothie (Chapter 9, Recipe 4)

Day 12:

- **Breakfast:** Green Detox Smoothie (Chapter 9, Recipe 1)
- **Lunch:** Minestrone Soup with White Beans and Pasta (Chapter 6, Recipe 6)
- **Dinner:** Spinach Strawberry Salad with Balsamic Glaze (Chapter 6, Recipe 3)
- **Snack:** Coconut Chia Seed Pudding (Chapter 7, Recipe 4)

Day 13:

- **Breakfast:** Avocado Toast with Poached Egg (Chapter 1, Recipe 5)
- **Lunch:** Moroccan Spiced Chicken Skewers (Chapter 4, Recipe 4)
- **Dinner:** Lentil Bolognese with Whole Grain Penne (Chapter 3, Recipe 9)
- **Snack:** Hummus with Crudites (Chapter 2, Recipe 2)

Day 14:

- **Breakfast:** Blueberry Banana Smoothie (Chapter 1, Recipe 6)
- **Lunch:** Lentil and Vegetable Stew (Chapter 7, Recipe 1)

- **Dinner:** Lemon Garlic Herb Roast Chicken (Chapter 3, Recipe 6) with a side of Mexican Street Corn Salad (Chapter 6, Recipe 9)
- **Snack:** Dark Chocolate Covered Strawberries (Chapter 8, Recipe 1)

Day 15:

- **Breakfast:** Quinoa Breakfast Bowl with Nuts and Seeds (Chapter 1, Recipe 9)
- **Lunch:** Tomato Basil Soup with Parmesan Crisps (Chapter 7, Recipe 2)
- **Dinner:** Beef and Broccoli Stir-Fry (Chapter 4, Recipe 5)
- **Snack:** Guacamole with Baked Tortilla Chips (Chapter 2, Recipe 1)

Day 16:

- **Breakfast:** Sweet Potato Hash with Turkey Sausage (Chapter 1, Recipe 10)
- **Lunch:** Chicken and Rice Soup (Chapter 7, Recipe 3)
- **Dinner:** Greek Salad with Feta and Olives (Chapter 6, Recipe 2)

- **Snack:** Almond Butter Energy Balls (Chapter 2, Recipe 10)

Day 17:

- **Breakfast:** Berry Sorbet (Chapter 8, Recipe 6)
- **Lunch:** Spicy Black Bean Soup (Chapter 7, Recipe 7)
- **Dinner:** Grilled Mahi-Mahi with Pineapple Salsa (Chapter 5, Recipe 2) served with a side of Greek Salad with Feta and Olives (Chapter 6, Recipe 2)
- **Snack:** Lemon Blueberry Yogurt Cake (Chapter 8, Recipe 9)

Day 18:

- **Breakfast:** Pumpkin Pie Bites (Chapter 8, Recipe 7)
- **Lunch:** Creamy Mushroom Soup (Chapter 7, Recipe 9)
- **Dinner:** Moroccan Chickpea Stew (Chapter 7, Recipe 8)
- **Snack:** Stuffed Mini Bell Peppers (Chapter 2, Recipe 8)

Day 19:

- **Breakfast:** Chocolate Avocado Mousse (Chapter 8, Recipe 8)
- **Lunch:** Butternut Squash and Apple Soup (Chapter 7, Recipe 4)
- **Dinner:** Lemon Dill Baked Halibut (Chapter 5, Recipe 6) with a side of Greek Salad with Feta and Olives (Chapter 6, Recipe 2)
- **Snack:** Greek Yogurt Popsicles with Fresh Berries (Chapter 8, Recipe 3)

Day 20:
- **Breakfast:** Oatmeal Raisin Energy Balls (Chapter 8, Recipe 10)
- **Lunch:** Thai Coconut Curry Soup (Chapter 6, Recipe 5)
- **Dinner:** Asian Turkey Lettuce Wraps (Chapter 3, Recipe 8)
- **Snack:** Peanut Butter Banana Protein Smoothie (Chapter 7, Recipe 4)

Day 21:
- **Breakfast:** Green Detox Smoothie (Chapter 9. , Recipe 1)

- **Lunch:** Minestrone Soup with White Beans and Pasta (Chapter 7, Recipe 6)
- **Dinner:** Spinach Strawberry Salad with Balsamic Glaze (Chapter 6, Recipe 3)
- **Snack:** Coconut Chia Seed Pudding (Chapter 8, Recipe 4)

Day 22:

- **Breakfast:** Avocado Toast with Poached Egg (Chapter 1, Recipe 5)
- **Lunch:** Moroccan Spiced Chicken Skewers (Chapter 4, Recipe 4)
- **Dinner:** Lentil Bolognese with Whole Grain Penne (Chapter 3, Recipe 9)
- **Snack:** Hummus with Crudites (Chapter 2, Recipe 2)

Day 23:

- **Breakfast:** Blueberry Banana Smoothie (Chapter 1, Recipe 6)
- **Lunch:** Lentil and Vegetable Stew (Chapter 7, Recipe 1)

- **Dinner:** Lemon Garlic Herb Roast Chicken (Chapter 4, Recipe 7) with a side of Mexican Street Corn Salad (Chapter 6, Recipe 9)
- **Snack:** Dark Chocolate Covered Strawberries (Chapter 8, Recipe 1)

Day 24:

- **Breakfast:** Quinoa Breakfast Bowl with Nuts and Seeds (Chapter 1, Recipe 9)
- **Lunch:** Tomato Basil Soup with Parmesan Crisps (Chapter 7, Recipe 2)
- **Dinner:** Beef and Broccoli Stir-Fry (Chapter 4, Recipe 5)
- **Snack:** Guacamole with Baked Tortilla Chips (Chapter 2, Recipe 1)

Day 25:

- **Breakfast:** Sweet Potato Hash with Turkey Sausage (Chapter 1, Recipe 10)
- **Lunch:** Chicken and Rice Soup (Chapter 7, Recipe 3)
- **Dinner:** Greek Salad with Feta and Olives (Chapter 6, Recipe 2)

- **Snack:** Almond Butter Energy Balls (Chapter 2, Recipe 10)

Day 26:

- **Breakfast:** Berry Sorbet (Chapter 8, Recipe 6)
- **Lunch:** Spicy Black Bean Soup (Chapter 7, Recipe 7)
- **Dinner:** Grilled Mahi-Mahi with Pineapple Salsa (Chapter 5, Recipe 2) served with a side of Greek Salad with Feta and Olives (Chapter 6, Recipe 2)
- **Snack:** Lemon Blueberry Yogurt Cake (Chapter 8, Recipe 9)

Day 27:

- **Breakfast:** Pumpkin Pie Bites (Chapter 8, Recipe 7)
- **Lunch:** Creamy Mushroom Soup (Chapter 7, Recipe 9)
- **Dinner:** Moroccan Chickpea Stew (Chapter 7, Recipe 8)
- **Snack:** Stuffed Mini Bell Peppers (Chapter 2, Recipe 8)

Day 28:

- **Breakfast:** Chocolate Avocado Mousse (Chapter 8, Recipe 8)
- **Lunch:** Butternut Squash and Apple Soup (Chapter 6, Recipe 4)
- **Dinner:** Lemon Dill Baked Halibut (Chapter 5, Recipe 6) with a side of Greek Salad with Feta and Olives (Chapter 6, Recipe 2)
- **Snack:** Greek Yogurt Popsicles with Fresh Berries (Chapter 8, Recipe 3)

Day 29:

- **Breakfast:** Oatmeal Raisin Energy Balls (Chapter 8, Recipe 10)
- **Lunch:** Thai Coconut Curry Soup (Chapter 7, Recipe 5)
- **Dinner:** Asian Turkey Lettuce Wraps (Chapter 3, Recipe 7)
- **Snack:** Peanut Butter Banana Protein Smoothie (Chapter 9, Recipe 4)

Day 30:

- **Breakfast:** Green Detox Smoothie (Chapter 9, Recipe 1)

- **Lunch:** Minestrone Soup with White Beans and Pasta (Chapter 7, Recipe 6)
- **Dinner:** Spinach Strawberry Salad with Balsamic Glaze (Chapter 6, Recipe 3)
- **Snack:** Coconut Chia Seed Pudding (Chapter 8, Recipe 4)

CONCLUSION

This book offers not just a diet plan, but a lifestyle change. It's about empowering yourself, taking control of your health, and embracing a new way of eating that can transform not just your body, but your entire well-being.

As you've learned throughout this book, intermittent fasting is not a one-size-fits-all approach. It's about finding what works best for you, listening to your body, and making sustainable changes that you can maintain for the long term.

By incorporating the delicious recipes, meal plans, and tips provided in this book, you're not just embarking on a journey to improve your physical health, but also your mental clarity, emotional well-being, and overall quality of life.

Remember, it's never too late to make a positive change. Whether you're looking to lose weight, boost your energy levels, or simply feel better in your skin, intermittent fasting can be a powerful tool to help you achieve your health goals.

So, as you close this book and embark on your intermittent fasting journey, do so with confidence, knowing that you have the knowledge, the tools, and the strength within you to succeed. Here's to a healthier, happier you!

COMPREHENSIVE TABLE OF CONTENTS

THANK YOU FOR

READING

Printed in Great Britain
by Amazon

45614418R00076